PORNOGRAPHY AND MASTURBATION ADDICTION MASTERY

A 7 STEP COMPREHENSIVE RECOVERY GUIDE TO RE-FOCUSING YOUR SEXUAL ENERGY, RETAINING YOUR SEED AND REBUILDING YOUR LIFE

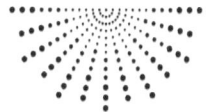

DAVID WHITEHEAD

SILK PUBLISHING

INTRODUCTION

Have you ever stopped to think about how lucky you are to be alive right now in this day and age? Never before in the history of humankind have we had so much raw *potential* at our disposal. The sheer amount of knowledge and influence we hold in our fingertips was once upon a time unfathomable, but now—thanks to technology—we hardly think about it at all. Perhaps this has always been the problem with us humans. *The excess*. The unsatiable need for more of it. How casually we quench that thirst until the cup runs dry. Life is littered with these traps of excess, and we have never been more efficient at fulfilling that need for more.

Cue the buzz word of the day: Addiction. You might have heard of it. It's a secret hiding in plain sight. You might have even learned about it from an early age, plastered on posters lining school hallways in big blocky letters overtop images of a spoon, a baggie, a tweaked-out mugshot of a scabbed-face man or woman. *Disgusting*, you might have thought to your middle school self. At that age, things like meth and heroine seem so alien. The concept of throwing your life away over a bottle of painkillers or booze simply did not compute. At

INTRODUCTION

least, that's how I felt when I was that age. But even then, as I was learning to look past the posters on my way to class, I had already planted the early seeds of my own addiction to masturbation and pornography.

Before we get too far ahead of ourselves, let's be clear; Masturbation, as an act alone, is absolutely normal. Feeling horny is normal. Wanting to cum is normal. There hasn't been a time on earth when human beings did not engage in the act of pleasuring themselves, and for a 13-year-old boy going through puberty, the act is almost inevitable. I don't hate myself for discovering masturbation when I did. I was the same as anyone else that age discovering their body. But overtime, I would learn to hate myself for over-indulging in the habit. I would learn to hate who I had become all for the sake of reaching climax, my deepening addiction to the pleasure, and for the sheer amount excess which had taken over my life.

For the longest time, I was sure that my masturbation habit, was just that—a habit—and nothing more. I remember feeling relieved when I found out how commonplace it was. Any time a friend or a television show alluded to it or made a joke about doing it, I thought to myself, *okay—see? It's perfectly normal. Nothing to see here. Carry on.*

That would have been true, perhaps back when I was thirteen. Jerking off once a day or every other day would have been fine. But to still be doing it every day 5 years later, or even ten? The picture begins to change. The jokes become a little less funny. To be in your twenties, jerking off multiple times a day, feeling the urge to do it every time you sit down at a computer. To still do it every single day even while being in a relationship, to even choose masturbating over sex itself. Is that normal?

For the longest time I never considered answering that question. My addiction had already taken hold long before I was ever ready to admit it. Porn had become a pillar of my life, too essential to tear down—too big to fail. It wasn't until I tried to quit and couldn't that I realized I had a problem. Porn had become more than just "a thing" it was something I needed. It had wormed itself into every aspect of my life and was warping it into something that, eventually, I hated.

I hated my life and I hated myself for being a slave to this habit—this disgusting excess. I had become the scabby listless face on the posters lining the hallway. I was a tweaker living solely for the next high that came from edging myself on to orgasm. Nothing else ever felt as good as that feeling of release, and soon I began sacrificing everything else to chase the high. Porn became the priority, and friends, family, hobbies, dreams, ambitions—all fell by the wayside. I burrowed myself deep within the habit and built my world completely around my need to cum. Whatever dream of a life I had envisioned for myself was disappearing in the margins. All that great potential I had was spent and forgotten.

I knew that I wanted more for myself than just porn. I wanted to be more, see more, do more. I wanted to have friends, fall in love, be successful, but porn was the only thing that my addicted mind would allow me to have. It suffocated me, tormented me, and for the longest time I secretly fed that desire until there was nothing else left. I was a shambolic robot running through the day-to-day motions, living from orgasm to orgasm, while the rest of my life passed me by. I wanted to change, but the addiction kept me glued tight to the very thoughts and behaviors it had invented to maintain itself. It wasn't until I started treating my excessive masturbation habits like the addiction that it really was, that I could even begin to find a way out of the pit I had fallen in.

If you have fallen into the same trap of pornography addiction, then I am glad to meet you here at the beginning of your new and improved life. I hope that my experiences as a recovering addict will be of some use to you and that together we can overcome the insatiable need for more as we return to a life of moderation and normalcy. If you are not currently suffering from this addiction and are reading this book as a means to understand what a friend or family member might be going through, I hope that you will gain some insight to how this addiction manifests itself and how you can support your loved ones who may be suffering in silence.

1

WHAT IS PORN AND MASTURBATION ADDICTION?

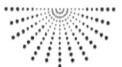

Masturbation, along with pornography and addiction are not uncommon terms. Yet, there still seems to be an overwhelming dissonance between the trio, at least when in terms of their public perception. There are many people who are prepared to tell you why masturbation, and masturbating to pornography, is not an addiction similar to drinking or using prescription painkillers. In a way, those arguing against porn and masturbation as addiction make good points about their distinctions from the other common addictions.

COMPARING ADDICTIONS

More "accepted" forms of addiction are the ones you ingest through the mouth or inject through a vein. You have to admit that the notion of putting something in your body that doesn't belong there really does capture that feeling of malice and malignancy that encapsulates addiction. Similarly, having your mind altered by the foreign substance, changing the very chemistry of your brain in such a way that it will affect you in the long term is little more straightforward to understand and is terrifying to watch unfold.

I'll never forget the first time I realized a good friend of mine was truly an alcoholic. It had happened a while after I met him, and funny enough, after months of regular nights out drinking after work. The particular time that struck me came one weekend I finally visited his apartment for the first time. His apartment was small, and bare, but fairly clean for a young single adult male—all save for one room, which I think he meant to close off. But the door was not shut all the way, and through half foot of space between the door and the frame, I could make out a room that was covered in empty bottles of various shapes and sizes.

When I say covered, I mean absolutely covered. The floor, the desk, atop the wardrobe, and lining the window frame. I must have gasped when I saw it, and quickly looked to see if he knew that I'd seen. Thankfully he hadn't, because I really wouldn't've known what to say. In fact, I didn't say anything for the longest time. I felt guilty, like I had accidentally stared into the man's soul. It wasn't until a mutual friend of ours actually had the courage to say something to him that it finally came out.

Perhaps I was too scared to confront him about his problem, because I wasn't ready to process my own gradual slip into addiction. Back then, I was eager to draw the line between his habit and mine. I assured myself that his thing and my thing were nothing alike, and that I was nowhere near as far deep into my own addiction than he was into his. At that point, I believed that my porn obsession was maybe a little excessive, but nothing too serious. It wasn't costing me anything other than time and I was able to convince myself that it would never cost me anything more than that. Of course, that's what the addicted mind tells you when you're staring at a projection of things to come.

That was my first true exposure to someone else's addiction, and it was the first time I realized how viscerally addiction could take over one's life. For the longest time, I kept coming back to that visual of the room covered in empty bottles, and now in retrospect, it makes sense why it resonated so much with me. It could have been a warning of things to come, but back then I was sure that wasn't me—that it could've never be me.

So, I can see why so many people are quick to point out how addiction to alcohol and pills are not on the same level as an addiction to pornography and masturbation. Perception plays an important role in how different addictions are treated by the masses, and perhaps one of the reasons why masturbation and pornography addiction do not get the same kind of recognition as other common addictions is because masturbation is a private, intimate act. This does not lend itself to the boisterous kind of fanfare that alcoholism or the opioid epidemic receives. When someone continually drinks or uses hard drugs, it is much more apparent to witness, and when we witness someone's spiral into drug or alcohol addiction, we are much more inclined to call it a problem. When we observe someone slowly give into their addiction to drugs or alcohol, it makes the malice all the more real. Consider how drastically methamphetamines affect the appearance of a regular user's face. Or how excessive alcohol use can make a normal adult human act like a belligerent child. These changes are easy to observe, and we are more likely to recognize addiction when the problem is on public display.

The opioid epidemic in particular, is currently gaining a lot of attention from the media because of how rampant the problem has spread across the country, but also because how easy it is to spot the afflicted opioid users who are having their entire lives upturned by their addiction. Masturbation, on the other hand, mostly occurs on the individual's own time, in the privacy of their own home. You wouldn't be able to point out a porn addict on the street, and it is much harder to pin down the difference between a "normal porn user" and a person who is suffering from pornography addiction.

HOW PORN ADDICTION WORKS

Although addiction to pornography is not as apparent as some of the other recognized addictions, it still has the capacity to do harm, and should be treated seriously. In America, pornography usage is widely popular. Over 40 million Americans classify themselves as regular porn users and about 200,000 people have admitted to having some level of addiction to masturbation and pornography consumption in America and out of that number, 10% have admitted being unsuccessful in their attempts to quit. By comparison, 20% of Americans consider themselves regular (binge) drinkers, and about 7% of drinkers are classified as having Alcohol Use Disorder. While not as prevalent as drinking, or some other types of addiction, pornography affects a similar percentage of regular users. As pornography becomes more attainable, one could expect these numbers to rise in term.

Perhaps as more people fall into the trap of porn addiction, more attention will be paid to the severity it poses. For those who are already suffering from the effects of pornography addiction, this recognition may be too little too late. Porn usage has been noted to seriously alter the perceptions of sex and pleasure. When you engage in the act of masturbation with pornography, your body learns to approach sex, and physical pleasure in a way that does not align with reality. In turn, this can cause physical issues whenever a porn addict engages in sexual activity.

Even more notable than the physical effects of frequent pornography usage are the mental manipulation it can weigh over the mind of the addicted. Pornography distorts sex, attraction, and intimacy in some of the worst ways possible. A lot of porn leans in on the warped idea that sex and pleasure is something immoral. This becomes a trope that is repeated over and over in porn's creation and portrayal. Many of the scenarios in erotica depict examples of cheating, impulsive behaviors, and general depravity which play on the sexual anxieties of its users.

The idea that if something feels right, then it is probably wrong, goes against the basis of sex being an intimate and consensual act that is aligned with the natural world. This distorted view of sex and pleasure can seriously affect the perception of regular porn users to the point where they cannot translate the acts of self-pleasure, with the act of sharing pleasure with another person. This eventually will create conflict in the relationships shared by that person. Their views towards sex, and members of the opposite sex can eventually be corrupted to the point where the afflicted are unable to distinguish the line between reality and fantasy.

THE CONTRADICTING PERCEPTIONS OF PORNOGRAPHY

One of the greatest obstacles which prevents us from taking pornography seriously is the normalization that has occurred since porn's rise in accessibility and acceptability. In popular culture, porn has become a staple of the young adult experience. Masturbation has become a common recreational act, similar to that of drinking or smoking. Now there is more media that is willing to discuss porn openly, and even feature porn as a form of artistic and creative expression (i.e., Game of Thrones). While the normalization of pornography could be perceived as a positive for sex culture, it still presents a challenge for millions of people who could possibly fall into the trap of excess presented by pornography and become addicted.

Another obstacle that faces those afflicted with pornography addiction, is the treatment of porn by more religious groups. For many prominent religions, sex is something that is sacred, and shared between two people for the purpose of procreation. When people are faces with the affliction of porn addiction, they are usually met with an overreaction by the religious institutions, who are quick to group pornography along with what they believe as a greater corruption of sexuality. Alcoholism and drug use used to be widely met in a similar fashion. Addiction was once treated as a kind of personal failure which needed to be corrected, instead of being a serious affliction beyond the cognition of the addict. Over the years, society has softened its views of addiction to drugs and alcohol, and now it is more common to see people "treated" from these addictions, rather than being "morally corrected."

Unfortunately, addiction to pornography hasn't yet earned this same kind of perception at large. Half of the population is ready to tell you why pornography is part of a healthy sexual identity, while the other half is ready to condemn you for even considering sex outside the confines of marriage. This results in the addict being faced with two extremes: either unchecked excessive pornography that is encouraged by secularized sex-positive culture, or complete abstention promoted by religious institutions. It's for this reason why pornography is such a devastating addiction. Without any proper mediation or advocacy for the problems posed by pornography, the addict is left to their own devices.

THE DANGERS OF A PRIVATE HABITUAL ADDICTION

The already private act of masturbation becomes even more privatized. The addiction occurs silently for years and years, creating the perfect storm. The effects of the addiction will often times go unnoticed, but whenever they manifest themselves, it usually occurs in devastating fashion—destroying relationships, causing divorce, separation, and worse still. At the very least, the addict will find themselves stuck on the path of unfulfillment, constantly chasing an increasingly fleeting feeling, until they are left as hollowed out husk of who they used to be.

For those on the outside, this may seem a little bit dramatic. But for anyone who has suffered from pornography addiction, or any addiction in general, will recognize the truth of the matter. When addiction takes a hold of your life, it changes you in profound ways. The science behind addiction points to the brain, which is altered by the continual habit. In some cases, such as drinking or ingesting drugs, the introduction of a new mind-altering substance creates can create a desire, a craving for more. In other cases, such as gambling or pornography, the alteration is self-generated. A boost of dopamine that courses through the brain and rewarding the action, creating the muscle-memory to do it again and again. No matter what causes it, addiction really boils down to the mind craving more.

This craving is a powerful force that has ruined the lives of millions across the globe. Now more than ever, we live in a time in our history where we have nearly unlimited access to food, alcohol, drugs, and porn. Unfortunately, this unchecked excess creates the perfect storm for addiction to occur. We can indulge ourselves to exuberant lengths, and in ways before we could've never thought possible. Our base reaction to the excess is positive. "More is better" after all, or is it? Without the ability to moderate how much we consume, we come perilously close to falling into the pitfalls of excess and addiction.

It is essential that we begin treating pornography as a serious addiction and begin considering ways to responsibly portray self-pleasure in a way that advocates for moderation. If we continue to confine sex and attraction exclusively in terms of its restriction and liberation, we will only continue to lose more people to addiction. I was one of those lost souls, stuck in purgatory somewhere between the abstinence I promised to my Christian upbringing and the sexual liberation that was promised to me by modernity. Being trapped between worlds did not help me find a healthy relationship with sex or self-pleasure, and in many ways helped shaped many of the mechanisms that prevented me from coming to terms with my addiction.

Only through speaking out and opening up the dialogue about pornography addiction can we ever hope to make progress in changing the public perception of masturbation and porn addiction. We need to have valuable conversations about the science and psychology behind pornography consumption. We need to try and better understand how this addiction manifests itself, and where it originates from. In my personal experience with pornography addiction, it wasn't until I really started analyzing my past history of masturbation and the thoughts and feelings I had associated with the act, that I began to understand why I had fallen into the pit in the first place. Once I opened up to myself about the reasons why I became addicted, I was able to confront the problems in my life that needed to change so that I could overcome and start living the life that I wanted to live.

2

HOW PORN AND MASTURBATION ADDICTION DEVELOPS

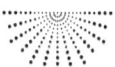

In this section, we will explore how pornography addiction begins, and how the act of masturbation is gradually transformed into an excessive habit with dire consequences. The best way to consider this, or any type of addiction, is like a continuation down a path. You may be at any point along this path, but you should pay close attention to the later stages of the addiction, and the serious impacts it can have on your life and relationships with others.

If you are reading this and are not an addict yourself, consider this section as a way to better understand and a person who is suffering from pornography addiction in your life. Hopefully giving my own personal perspective and experience with masturbation addiction can help you empathize with what an addict might currently be going through and help you aid in their recovery.

HOW PORN ADDICTION BEGINS

As noted in previous sections, masturbation is a normal act which a large percentage of people engage in regularly. For most, masturbation begins in the early stages of puberty as the developing mind and body of the teenager becomes more likely to explore these changes firsthand. In my personal experience, I was almost thirteen years old when I first started touching myself and like many during their first time, I did not understand exactly what had happened.

I was fortunate growing up in a family that had money, and so I was naturally spoiled with my own room, TV, game system, and personal laptop. Also, as the oldest child, I was often left to my own devices, as my parents were busy keeping up with the demands of my younger siblings. On one such night, after I was sure everyone was asleep, I turned on the TV and flipped through the seemingly infinite amount of channels offered by satellite TV. It should be noted that I grew up in a protestant Christian household, and both of my parents did as much as you might expect to ensure that I upheld my purity. However, at that age it didn't take much to feed my growing interest in the female anatomy. I remember landing on a spring break special on MTV, and the rest was history.

When I discovered masturbation, it felt immediately like I had done something wrong. I remember feeling mortified by the stain I had created beneath my sheets and took extra care to make sure I was the one who ended up washing them to avoid my parents finding out. At the same time, however wrong it might have felt, I was also caught up in the rush of excitement and build up it created in me. That feeling of inching towards climax was unlike anything I had experienced up to that point in my life. So, I found myself constantly thinking about how I could recreate that sensation.

It didn't take long for me to realize after that first incident that I basically had the entirety of the internet at my disposal to help recreate that moment. So, out came the laptop sitting on top of my bed comforter, bright screen emanating in my dark bedroom. My first engagements with porn started very tamely. Googling words such as boobs, and naked (safe search off) was my first introduction and did plenty to stimulate the first few times.

I was naïve then, but still clever enough to know how to hide it from my parents and quickly learned how to erase the lewd searches from my browser history, and even went as far as deleting every cookie and keystroke from my laptop each time I went on my nightly binges. Even then, I remember lying awake in bed after I had cleaned up and tucked my laptop away, staring up at my ceiling and thinking about what I had done and what it all meant. The second and third time still felt as good as the first, and I couldn't believe how easy it was to create that feeling. Just my hand and a couple of pixelated images of breasts and ass. My mind raced between feelings of pleasure and guilt, and I found myself split between planning out my next orgasm and running through a list of reasons why I should never touch myself again.

In the early stages of my masturbation habit, I was compelled by the positive feelings it created whenever I engaged in the process of masturbation. The search for porn itself became an integral part of the process, and part of my reward. I began following the links associated with the images and was directed to blogs and webpages dedicated to different porn actresses and categories. It felt like my curiosity was being constantly rewarded and I found newer and better means to fulfill that need to masturbate.

This process of searching, finding, and rewarding myself became a continual cycle that largely shaped the full progression of my pornography addiction. After moving from Google image search to actual websites, I discovered actual videos which amplified the reward, and propelled me further into the habit. Ironically, the feelings of guilt and remorse that were always present after the fact also contributed to the cycle continuing on. Perhaps if I were a little less worried about the consequences of my actions, and a little more foolhardy in my approach to masturbating, I would have been caught early on by my parents, which could have radically changed how my habit progressed. But instead, I was clever and conscious about my actions. So, it became an exercise of stealth. I was always careful not to draw the attention of my parents, and without their reprimand, I gave myself the greenlight to carry on.

The more comfortable I grew in the process, the more regular it became part of my daily routine. I would "have" to cum at least once a day to feel satiated, but sometimes I felt the urge creeping up a second or a third time. I found myself pulling out my laptop whenever a chance for privacy presented itself. Anytime my mother and father were out of the house, I would quickly go through the process and try to rub one off before either of them was able to check on me. I discovered that the riskier times I jerked off, the more it added to the excitement. In hindsight, this should have been the earliest warning to myself that my masturbation habit was escalating towards an addiction.

Without any kind of seminal event that broke the cycle, it was able to progress for years and years without interruption. For the longest time, the effects didn't seem to be all that bad. I was a regular porn consumer for just about every day during my middle and high school years. The only noticeable negative during this time was the amount of time I spent searching for porn and masturbating. Once I started dating and becoming more sexually active in high school, I also noticed that my interest in pornography declined, and I took this as a sign that I really didn't have a problem. But surely enough, the masturbation and the porn did not stop, and after a while of being in a relationship I found it more appealing to fall back on my habit, whenever it offered the promise of something a little more exciting.

Naturally, this created a few problems in some of my early relationships. I wasn't aware of it at the time, but porn was creating a warped image of sexuality and intimacy which was completely out of the norms of reality. I was cultivating an unconscious expectation for my partners and believed that our physical intimacy to resemble the erotic videos I consumed, but of course reality always fell short.

This naturally leads into the next section, which I like to call:

HOW PORN ADDICTION INFLUENCES RELATIONSHIPS

Growing up, I always wanted to have a relationship that mirrored my parents. From my perspective, they were perfect for each other and had a strong and healthy dependance on one another, which was easy to see and feel when living under their roof. Whenever I started taking an interest in the opposite sex, it was always through the frame of trying to find "the one" and I heavily romanticized this idea. I was deeply invested in the search for true love, similar to what my parents had, and much of time that wasn't spent doing schoolwork, sports, or indulging in bad habits, was spent pursuing the next love of my life. Which, of course was ridiculous in hindsight.

For one, I was deeply immature and had no real idea of what love really meant. I had only seen the surface of deep and intimate love that was shared by my parents. So how could I have possibly known if what I felt was ever that kind of love. Additionally, I was putting far too much emphasis on something which should have developed naturally over a period of time. I wasn't allowing myself to fully explore my interests or try to figure out who I really was as a person. I had settled on the idea that I needed to find love as soon as possible, so that I could recreate the intimacy and love shared by mom and dad.

But thirdly, and perhaps worst of all, the whole time I was romanticizing love and pursuing the perfect relationship, I was engaging in the complete opposite when it came to sex and physical intimacy. Unintentionally, I had separated sex and love to the point where they became virtually incompatible. Sex had become this act of self-pleasure, with hints of sin and depravity. Self-pleasure had become something that was innately wrong, sinful. This was partly due to growing up in a religious household, but the rest came from my own innate desire to be upstanding in the eyes of my family and friends. In public, I wanted to shape this identity of a good person without any flaws and or shortcomings.

This resulted in me suppressing many of the habits, thoughts, and behaviors that could have negatively affected other's perception of me. Masturbation was not good Christian behavior, and therefore I went to great lengths to make sure that my family never knew that I masturbated or regularly looked at pornography. I went as far as not really disclosing it with my friends either. Even we matured, and our jokes and conversations shifted to topics of sex, attraction, and masturbation. I always felt like treading water in these situations and never shared that side of me. And of course, it never came up in the long, deep, "intimate" conversations with the girls I was seriously dating at the time. Sex, and sexual pleasure, was something private—exclusively to me. This however was a direct contradiction to what sex and physical intimacy really was: something shared between two people

Pornography had allowed me an outlet to explore, and in

many ways, shape my sexual interests. After years of masturbating, I had developed particular interests in different body types of women and various scenarios which were slowly extending beyond the reach of reality. I would watch a porn video that featured a threesome and fantasize about being with two women at the same time, even though that went against everything that I wanted to have in an actual romantic relationship. I was trying to find a partner to build a life together with, while I was also furiously beating my dick to hardcore squirt videos.

The contradiction between these two areas of love that I was trying to fulfill was becoming too large to sustain itself. From high school to college, my relationships suffered because of this. The girls I wanted to be with, I held in a different light. They became embodiments of this ideal of what a romantic partner should be like, and I had no idea how to merge this image of them to the image of what I believed sex and pleasure to be. It's not that they didn't live up to the expectations I had developed towards sex, but they simply could not allow them to exist that space. They didn't belong there. They didn't fit into this warped reality I had created around sex and pleasure. I wanted to be intimate with them, but my mind would not let them into that space I had cultivated for so long.

That space was mine—It was for me and the porn, and every living, breathing, human that ever wanted to be physically close with me found themselves unable to connect with me in the way we both wanted to. I didn't figure this out the first or the second time. It took me lots hard breakups, emotional words, and tears before I began to realize that something was wrong with me, and it took me even longer to admit that a big part of the problem was my advancing addiction to pornography.

I went through heartbreak after heartbreak over this wall

I had created around myself—The great wall of porn, which had cut me off from true physical attachment. When I met the girl of my dreams in college, I wanted nothing else in the world than to be with her. Our relationship sprang to life almost spontaneously. Once we started talking, everything fell into place naturally. We were a perfect fit for each other in almost every single way, and we became intimately close. We poured out our hearts for each other and fell deeply in love. Hours with her felt like minutes, and I was positive she was "the one" after all these years of searching. We were together for several months, seriously dating, and deeply in love with each other, but whenever things began to get physical between us two, the cracks began to show, and eventually—we fell apart.

At this point in my early to mid-twenties, I had been a regular porn user for about ten years. Ten years of walling myself off and creating this warped reality of sex as this sinful, secluded act. After ten years of muddying the waters of intimacy with these over-indulgent fantasies of threesomes, orgies, and BDSM, I had no idea where the real thing was supposed to fit in. I had cultivated a garden of weeds and left no room for a flower. How could deep emotional love fit into this world of depravity I had created for sex. There was no way to make it work.

And that's why I couldn't get a boner. Performance issues, at twenty-two. Not because of anything physically wrong with me, but because I was in this foreign headspace. How was I supposed to get off when there's another person here? Intimacy with another human being? Impossible. Unheard of. Even when I was with the love of my life, a woman who perfect in every single way—A gorgeous human being, someone who I was deeply physically attracted to, but I couldn't get hard for. I wasn't able to get into the moment because I loved her too much, and couldn't accept her into my concept of pleasure, which had been corrupted by porn.

As you can imagine, this was the ultimate downfall of the relationship. My girlfriend, who I was sure was going to one day be a fiancé and wife, was deeply confused and hurt by her inability to turn me on. We tried to work around it for a while, but each time we felt out love swell up to the point of physicality, we fell flat on our faces. At this point, I was frantic to find out what was wrong with me. I was suspicious that my porn habit could have been the culprit, but I was plagued by other ideas and theories behind our physical incompatibility, which winded up fueling a vicious cycle of insecurity and doubt.

I was worried that the problem was me in relation to my inadequacy, and instead of trying to figure out why there was a problem in the first place, I began obsessing over the rift it was causing. Soon, I was inundated with thoughts of our relationship falling apart, that it did just that. And we grew further and further apart, driven by that great wall, which with the help of insecurity and doubt, had expanded out by several rings. For many years, I was caught up in this sadness. I couldn't get over my failure to secure "the one" and live up to my parents' lofty relationship. I wasn't motivated in the slightest to try for a long time, and all the while I consoled myself with more masturbation, more porn, and more indulgence.

HOW PORN ADDICTION ADVANCES

Like any good addiction, pornography creates a habit that becomes so intrinsically engrained in your routine, it is impossible to shake. The result is a vicious cycle, designed to take you down further and further into your despair, creating the false notion that the only thing there is left to console you is the very source of the despair, so you keep drawing from that well until your reach rock bottom. This is where I was for a long period after breaking up with "the one," now referred to as "the one who got away."

I had convinced myself that I simply wasn't good enough for her. And I thought up of so many reasons for why that was so, but thanks to pornography, I believed it must have been because I was not enough for her. My insecurity drove me to believe that because I wasn't as big, or sexy as the guys in the videos I jerked off to, I wasn't able to pull it off with the girl of my dreams. I couldn't live up to the idea of sex that I had created in my head. And I hated myself for it and resigned to jerking off because that's all I believed I was capable of.

The thing about masturbation is that it physically good, and in the moment, your focus solely lies on that feeling of pleasure. During periods of depression, masturbation became a form of escape. It was a time when I wasn't plagued by thoughts of my failures or inadequacies. It was just about feeling good, and the buildup to a dopamine hit, that made every other bad feeling melt away. But surely enough, after each orgasm there came a period of heightened awareness, followed swiftly by disgust, self-loathing, and a resigned slump back into depression.

This depression, which highlighted my loneliness and feelings of inadequacy, extended to other areas of my life. Whenever I was feeling low, I felt like an absolute failure in everything I attempted. School, work, and physical fitness fell by the wayside and I started to compound my depression and addiction to pornography with other overindulgences. I was eating more junk food than ever; ordering take out just about every night and always treating myself with ice cream and chocolates. I gained more and weight during this period, which only increased my negative self-image and demotivated me from pursuing other romantic partners, or even going out and spending time with friends.

I was slowly becoming antisocial, and the negative feelings I was developing towards myself was being reinforced by worsening physical health and my strained personal relationships with my friends and family. I chose to play videogames and binge hours of television instead of keeping up with schoolwork, or looking for a new job, and whenever I was bored with that, it was back to the porn. At my lowest points, I would masturbate two to three times each day, sometimes for hours at a time, looking for different videos and distracting myself with this alternate reality.

Years of masturbating to porn will create a certain level of tolerance towards what will and won't get you off. Similar to smoking, or drinking, or any other kind of addiction—you become dulled to the sensations, and so you need more stimulation in order to reach the same heights of ecstasy as you felt the first time you started using. With porn, this occurs just the same, and so you try to find different content to fill that need. For me, I became more interested in the hardcore variants of pornography. In hindsight, it makes sense why I veered off into this direction. Pleasure, sex, and sin had always been synonymous to me, so the more sinful and debauched the videos, the more heightened the pleasure.

At this point of my depression, I was fully feeding my addiction to pornography, which in turn only exacerbated my depression even further. By doubling down on hardcore porn videos, I was moving further away from the wholesome physical intimacy that I wanted to share with another person. Whenever I attempted to date again, after losing "the one" I was still deeply affected by the unrealistic expectations of sex that I had invested in during my hardcore porn binges. I had developed a need for freaky sexual desires, but I was still conditioned to withhold that completely whenever I tried forming a physical relationship with another person, which only resulted in more disappointment, regret, and shame.

When dating failed me, I would come crawling back to the porn. Only this time, I needed more of it. I needed better quality videos, so I actually subscribed to different porn sites so I could access the full-length videos and high-definition quality. At this point my addiction had entered a new phase, it was not only costing me time or physical intimacy, but it was also affecting me financially.

THE FINANCIAL IMPACT OF PORN

Right around when I started paying for monthly subscriptions to different porn websites is when I really started to consider that I might be addicted to porn. I was paying close to $30 each month just to have access to better quality videos. However, the real financial impact wouldn't come until I discovered that many of these big porn sites also offered cam-girl services.

For those who are not aware, these webcam services are just another cog in the massive porn industry. Girls from all over the world create an account and perform various lewd acts live, in front of paying clients. The sites that host these interactions get a cut from the "private" interactions that occur between the performer and the client. The cost for these interactions is not cheap either. Models typically will charge three to four dollars a minute for a private cam show. For some perspective, these shows can last however long the client wishes, but even if you were to engage in a private show for only a handful of minutes, you could expect to pay upwards of twenty to thirty dollars per show.

The truly alarming thing about these cam-shows are that there doesn't have to be any upward limit to how long you spend in a private chat, or how much you spend on a single interaction. For many of these sites, you only need to enter in your credit card information to gain access to all of the different cam models. With this open-ended kind of setup, it became perilously easy for me to spend $50 to $100 d0llars on a night of interacting with various models, paying for these interactions with a mouse-click and the meek promise offered by a high credit line.

Discovering cam shows devastated me financially. I would visit the cam sites just about every other day, and while I thought I was being frugal by only entering the chatrooms for a few minutes at a time, it was all adding up over time. I was spending hundreds of dollars a month that I simply did not have, and I had to take extra jobs working just to pay off these interactions which only lasted 5 to 10 minutes each. This made my porn addiction feel very real to me. Suddenly I was like the 5-pack a day smoker, or the weekend binge drinker budgeting just to maintain the habit. I realized that I had essentially become the sleazy guy that regularly visits the strip club, only I was doing it from behind a screen.

Shipping off a hundred dollars each month for porn only further impacted my social life in negative ways. If there ever was an opportunity to go somewhere or do something with my friends, I couldn't afford it. If I needed to buy something for my apartment, or wanted to splurge on some extra groceries, I was unable to splash out the cash. My addiction was limiting me, and reducing the overall value of my life, and continued to feed the negative cycle of depression. No money for real social interactions meant that my relationships with my friends and family were further strained.

I became the person who never was up for it. The flake. After a few times of not being able to make a social outing, friends stopped inviting me in the first place. I was more walled off than ever and did my best to hide what was going on to my friends and family. Living alone made that possible, and now that I was a college graduate and working adult, people just assumed I was toiling away and left me alone to do my own thing. But in truth, I wasn't toiling as much as I was just wasting my life. Wasting away in my dingy apartment, which was all I could afford, coming home after working a non-career job and spending the rest of my time watching TV and masturbating to porn.

THE VICIOUS CYCLE OF PORN ADDICTION

I had fallen into a pathetic routine, which was able to sustain itself for months, and it was all because of porn. I was living for the porn, and the heightened moments that came during the buildup to ejaculation. This became the only time I felt excited, or happy, or alive. Everything else was a black pit of despair. I would clean up after myself and immediately be reminded about all of the negative feelings I was trying to escape. The failures, the lost connections, the ruined relationships. It all came back at once and smothered me. These negative feelings kept me away from the ones I loved and made me believe that the only happiness on earth left for me was what I could watch from behind a screen.

I had surrendered my life to porn, and as a result, porn kept me tight in its clutches. After falling into debt paying off the credit cards, I had squandered on cam sites, I was working for porn, laboring for months to pay off the interest that had compounded on an orgasm which lasted only seconds. And after months of living and working for porn, what did I have to show for it? Absolutely nothing.

I was a loser. Deadbeat. Addict. I hated myself and who I had become. I would spend hours at night, staring up at the ceiling and wincing at the lost opportunities and failures. I constantly wondered what life could be like if I had never invested so much of my time and efforts into porn. I was so far away removed from that image of a person that I wanted to be growing up. I regretted just about everything I had done with my life, and worst of all, I was completely alone.

I would constantly think about my mother and father's relationship, that golden city on a hill. That model, I sought to recreate in my own life, and I would well up with tears and cry myself to sleep. Where in the world had that gone? Was that kind of love and intimacy even possible? In my deepest pit of despair, I could find no way to ever come close to that kind of life and love. I thought that it was truly impossible. I was positive in those moments, that I was incapable of it, and when assessing the carnage that was my life, I was there at the epicenter. Just me, my laptop, and my porn.

I hated myself. I truly did, and I was living a desolate and empty life. The cycle had funneled me down all the way to the bottom, and all that was left there was my shame. Shame, which for me was the single self-propelling momentum behind my spiraling pornography addiction. I had spent my entire life conflating pleasure and shame to the point where I wasn't able to find joy in anything. Porn: the root of my depression had become an affirmation that the only way I could ever be happy was being alone, but every fiber of my being longed for true connection. The contradiction within myself was tearing me apart.

3

A TIME TO HEAL: WHY YOU ARE READY TO QUIT PORN FOREVER

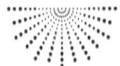

At my lowest, I was unable to reconcile the contradiction within. This inner conflict combusted into shame, which had propelled forward into this addiction, and left me choking in its fumes.

I cannot say with any certainty what might be the machine that drives your pornography addiction. Shame was mine. But just like with any other addiction, there could be any number of reasons why someone gets sent down the path. Your addiction is unique to your own journey, and even though the fuel might be different between us, the repair process is essentially the same. And yes, it's not too late to repair.

The first step to solving any problem, is recognizing that one is there in the first place. By reading this book, you are already on this step. You have realized that something is not right with your life, and your relationship with pornography and masturbation. You are recognizing that your relationship with sex has developed into something that is unnatural, and the simple act of self-pleasure has been corrupted to the point where it has taken the reigns of your entire life.

Now that you are able to see the problem that addiction has caused in your life, you are ready to enact real change. You were walking down the wrong path, but now you've stopped—paused for a moment to reassess. What you decide to do or not do in this moment could be the time when you finally turn it all around and lead yourself to greener pastures. It's in this moment now, that you must continue to press into raw and uneasy truth. Now is the time to really dig into your head and breakdown the cycle that has consumed your life so entirely. Once you are open to diving into the mechanics behind your addiction, you will be able to identify the source. Recognizing the negative feelings, trauma, or motivation that's behind your addiction is the first step to fixing the problem.

And do not feel discouraged by the fact that a problem is there. There's nothing wrong with being flawed. Everyone becomes broken in their own way and in their own time. Now is not the time for you to accept the reality of this moment, but to recognize all the things that could be. The life that you wanted before addiction before pornography took control over you, is still out there to be had, and you are not as far away from your perfect life as you might believe. You just need to repair your broken soul, replace the negative habits you have created for yourself, and keep chugging along until you reach the life you always wanted to live.

The beauty of the human soul is its incredible ability to heal itself. Even though you are broken now, you are still capable of recovering from your addiction. The healing will take time, but you will heal, and things will start to turn around. Your addiction has robbed you blind of the things in life that really matter to you. As you heal, you will learn to replace the stolen goods, and start rebuilding a life closer to the one you want to have. It won't always be easy, and the garden you cultivate wont always look pretty. There will be plenty of weeds that will continue to pop up through the cracks, but you're a gardener now. If you are ready to put on the gloves and get dirty, then you will be up for the toil.

PREPARING YOURSELF FOR THE BATTLE TO COME

Perhaps, gardening is too soft a metaphor for journey to recovery. If your journey is anything like mine, then it will be a full-on uphill battle. Addiction is a war with yourself, with guerilla warfare happening every day on the frontlines of your mind. There will be battles that you win, and battles that you lose. And if there was only one thing, I could teach you, it would be resilience. Because you will lose a battle or two, and when the war is against yourself, the losses can feel devastating. It's important to be resilient to the losses, the disappointments, the heart aches. You are in for an uphill battle, and it will not be easy. Your addicted mind is the enemy. It has become infected by your indulgence, and only cares about serving itself. It is ready to crush every bone in your body and turn your mind into a puddle of mush. You must be resilient. Your addiction is an enemy that must be stopped at all cost, and you are the only one who can lead the charge.

Resilience is the first lesson and having realistic expectations about the causalities of internal warfare will give you valuable perspective whenever you are inevitably handed defeats by the hand of your enemy. Your addicted mind is crafty. It understands you just as well as you understand yourself, if not better. It will use anything as ammunition to get what it wants, and it already knows all of your weaknesses. That is why it is equally important to bring in reinforcements for your war against addiction.

THE IMPORTANCE OF BUILDING COMMUNITY

Your addicted mind, however conniving it may be, has a weakness of its own. It will always only have itself. It is the source of your loneliness, remember? It would rather keep you cut off from every other living thing, just so it can milk you further to quench its insatiable thirst. When you are isolated and battling alone, the addicted mind will almost always win. You need to have outside reinforcements to help you turn the tide and reclaim your life from addiction.

If you're anything like me, then bringing in reinforcements will not be easy. The shame that propelled my addiction was equally as capable of keeping me from ever opening up to the people around me. My reaction was to always bottle up when it came to interacting with other people. I had to project this image of a flawless person, and I was afraid of ruining the façade. I had to fight my shame directly, hand to hand combat. I got down in the mud with my shame and my pride and force myself to open up, and even giving it my all I found it almost impossible to open up to my friends and family about my addiction to porn and masturbation.

I don't think I would have ever been able to open up, if not for an online community of recovering porn addicts, known widely as the No-Fap movement. Discovered by chance on Reddit, this community was my first introduction to others who shared my affliction. Being introduced to this community was essential to helping me learn how to communicate about my addiction as well as validate this war that I was trying to wage against myself.

What made the community so effective for me, was how honestly and openly the other members were able to communicate. They were an incredibly active group which posted around the clock, twenty-four-seven. There was also a wide diversity of users who came from all areas along the path of addiction. There were those who were new to process like me, and recovery veterans who did not hesitate to spill their wisdom and encouragement whenever they could.

Finding a group of people who faced the same struggles as myself, gave me incredible insight to the enemy. They taught me how my addicted mind works and gave me ideas on what strategies were needed to defeat my obsession with porn. But even with this constant barrage of support, I still needed to be able to reclaim the real-life connections I had with my friends and family. The No-Fap Community was wholesome, and pure, but there was still a level of disconnect there, as there will be with any exclusively online community. I still needed to tear down the great wall of shame that I built between me and the people I loved.

But the No-Fap community still helped in that regard, because even though I was interacting with online strangers, I was developing the all-important muscle memory to talk about my porn addiction. Being able to share with the community enabled me to grow more comfortable with expressing my addiction, and eventually I was able to overcome my pride and shame and share my inner conflicts with my friends and family.

Community is essential because it creates an environment of accountability. The addicted mind hates this word, and it fears the consequences of you having something else to live for. All your addiction will ever have at its disposal is porn, but you have everything else as possible ammunition. Now, your addiction is the one on the retreat, and the battles rage on, but you feel the tide start to turn.

Addiction won't end overnight, and even after bringing in reinforcements, it doesn't mean that victory is imminent. However, with every small victory you earn along the way, you will have reclaimed another piece of your life back. No matter how small your victories may be, you will start collecting them, and they will add up. Even as the war rages on, your small victories will eventually be enough to sustain you. They will make your resolve stronger. You will have more reasons to push on, even after you have faltered. You will learn to fall back on your growth and use your past victories to continue fighting the good fight. And eventually you will win.

A LOOK AHEAD AT THE VICTORIES TO COME

What waits for you is the promise of a better life. A life that is filled with real connections that matter. A relationship with sex that isn't corrupted by sin. A pathway to pleasure that is ignorant of shame. True bliss—this is what you are missing. It's still out there waiting for you. You can't see it yet, but it never went away. There is a way to feel complete and whole, and once you discover what truly fulfills your base needs, you won't need the porn anymore.

Once you believe in it, everything else will seem to fall into place. You will come to terms with the source of your addiction and will have healed it. Now everything that was closed off to you is suddenly open again. You don't have to be lonely anymore. There are people out there for you, who love you and accept you for who you are—flaws and all, because you are adequate. You are reason enough. Those dreams you have continue to be valid, so long as you feel compelled to reach, and even if you don't it will have still been enough. Life after addiction is so much sweeter than anything you could have ever imagined. It's all right there, are you ready to take it?

4

THE SEVEN CRUCIAL STEPS TO RECOVER FROM PORNOGRAPHY ADDICTION

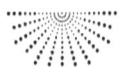

Now that you are ready to begin your journey towards recovery, here is the comprehensive guide to leaving your pornography addiction in your past, and paving a new, and better path forward. In the early days of recognizing my pornography addiction, I was hesitant to put any faith in the internet articles, and various help books which advocated for a complete recovery in just a handful of steps. At that point, I was fully aware of how thoroughly pornography had wrecked my entire life, and I was skeptical to seek out any kind of help using self-help blogs, or books.

I ended up fumbling through my recovery on my own. For the longest time, I wasn't interested at all for asking for help about my addiction, even when I felt it's full impact. The shame I felt in my own personal weakness kept me from extending an arm out for aid. I was defiantly trying to navigate the waters on my own, and while I am glad that I had the courage to crawl my way out of my addiction, I really wish I had the foresight to seek out help earlier on. Perhaps then, I would have found myself on the right path much sooner. But alas, I am here now, and I am glad to be the one to help you on your own path towards recovery.

My recovery did not happen according to any plan, and I wouldn't expect yours to either. Recovery doesn't happen linearly, and while these steps are presented in an order, do not feel like you are spinning wheels by moving from one to seven. All seven of these steps are moving in the right direction, and as long as you are moving forward down the right path, you are going to win battles down the road. In truth, these steps are all taken in tandem. You are supposed to take them all at once, and whenever you can. They are all designed to shepherd you away from the negative mentalities and behaviors which contributed to your addiction, and as long as you are at least attempting one, you are removing yourself further from the afflicted person who you were before.

This is the way I progressed at least, however not nearly as efficient. If anything, the order of these seven steps is arranged by the level of their effectiveness as it corresponds with where you are at in different stages of your recovery. Steps 1 through 3 are going to be extremely helpful for the beginning phases of your journey. By focusing on the earlier steps first, you will help build a better base to build the rest of your recovery on. Likewise, the later stages 6, and 7 are designed to be more reflective, which is most beneficial for the person who has been on the path of recovery for a longer time.

In the middle, you are left with steps 4 and 5, which are the constant behavioral actions which are essential at any stage of your recovery. These are the steps you should always strive for, but don't expect to make it far unless you have already established the first three steps.

The reflection and introspection that comes with the

final steps, hint at probably the hardest truth you can hear in the early stages of recovery; that is, that recovery is a continual process—one that has no end. You might be in a point in your life where this sounds like a resignation, but I cannot tell you how wrong you are. Now I get it, you want to be "cured" now. You don't want to ever feel as low as you do now. You want the recovery to be quick shot, a hard line. You want to be able to paint your life in completely different colors on either side of this decision to quit throwing away your life for porn. But this is not the truth. The truth is that life is in itself a continual process, and recovery is just another way of life.

Accepting that there is no magical cure for your pornography addiction and embracing the recovery lifestyle is essential to forming a positive relationship with the seven steps. You are a collection of many past selves. Your addicted mind is still a part of you and will remain there forever. Recovery is not about denying your addiction exists or forgetting about when it had complete control over you. Recovery is about recognizing that your addicted mind is just one of many sides you have to offer. You are a beautifully complex human being. You are born in three dimensions. You are not flat. These other sides to you have always been there, but addiction has smothered them in its hostile takeover. Now that you are coming to terms with your addiction to masturbation and pornography, you are ready to bring balance back to yourself, and reclaim your identity.

As I said before, your addiction recovery is like an ongoing battle with yourself. While its all-out warfare at the moment, this does not mean your future will always be full of casualties. There will be a time of peace for you, if you continue down the path of recovery. Someday you will be able to look back at the times when your life was out of control, and you will feel thankful for your own resilience when the war was raging. There may not be a magical cure, but there is a future out there for you. A future free from addiction to masturbation and pornography. It is going to be so much better than your present moment, you just need to keep fighting the good fight.

5

STEP 1: GETTING REAL WITH YOURSELF

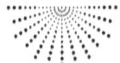

While these steps do not necessarily need to occur in a set order, you will find that addressing this first step will unlock many doors which can prove extremely helpful in the early stages of your addiction recovery. Now is the time for you to get real with yourself. To admit that you have a problem with porn. Up to this point, you have let your pornography obsession take control of your life. You have allowed porn to worm its way into how you pleasure yourself, the way you perceive yourself, and your intimacy with others.

Now is the time to wake up to the reality of the situation. You are not living your best possible life. You are in a pit. There are walls all around you, and they reach way above your head. You are isolated now, trapped in this obsession with porn. You never wanted this life for yourself. You never wanted to reduce yourself down to the singular moment of orgasm. You wanted more than that. Now you are neglecting the things in your life that really mattered to you, and there is no amount of convenience offered by porn that makes this one-dimensional existence okay. You once wanted to live a rich life, full of real stuff, things that mattered. You wanted real and raw emotions, and feelings, and love. You never wanted to resign to cold lifeless interactions with strangers. This is you not living up to your potential; this is fixation, indulgence, and squander.

This addiction is really just you hiding from something, whatever it is. Something deeper. You had a reason to drag yourself down here. Maybe you were scared. Maybe you were running away. Maybe you were hurt and just wanted to fold in on yourself and block out the rest of the world. You are not ready to face *it*, whatever it really is. Perhaps it's something deeper. It could be your hurt, your trauma, your insecurity, your loss, your broken heart. Maybe it's your shame holding it all together.

For me it was shame. Shame was the glue that kept me stuck to my addictive thought and behavior patterns. I was so ashamed by how far I had let my life get away from me, that I did not want to face the truth of the matter. I wanted to pretend like I was okay, that I was happy being impervious to the world around me. I was a person who did not want to admit fault, even to myself, and even when I was wandering around the wasteland of my own shortcomings. Each time I achieved a fleeting moment of release after ejaculation, it was quickly back to the process or suppressing the reality of my actions. I had to admit to myself that I really did just spent hours looking for a video to jerk off to or had spent hundreds of dollars that I didn't have just for shallow five-minute interactions with cam-girls. I couldn't even look at myself in the mirror, I was so ashamed.

In order to avoid this feeling of shame, I was quick to do whatever action was necessary to not let the self-disappointment sink into myself. I quickly busied myself with spending hours scrolling through social media, getting lost down YouTube rabbit holes, playing video games, or diving head-first into a dead-end hobby. But in reality, 9 times out of the 10 it was back to the incognito browser. Back to the self-destructive habit that I just couldn't get away from.

The shame I felt was immense, and it only ever grew and grew. I hated myself for being this way. Being so weak. So, vulnerability was never an option for me. I had to be hard, cold, detached. I would distract myself so I wouldn't have to face the reality of my actions, because I was so disappointed in myself, and it was through this distraction that my addiction was able to sustain itself for years.

My inability to face my own disappointment and shame myself kept me from ever addressing the shithole that I found myself in. I was truly living in denial, and it wasn't until I finally had the courage to face the reality of my situation, that I was able to figure out how to get myself out again.

What eventually changed was how I approached myself whenever I began to feel vulnerable. Vulnerability for me was the weak point being exploited by my addiction. Porn promised itself to be the ultimate distraction to keep me from plumbing the depths of my sadness. Porn had used this weak spot for years to convince me that the vulnerability was something that needed to be squashed and rebutted immediately. It wasn't until I started taking a chance with myself, that I started tor realize that vulnerability was not a liability, but a different kind of affirmation to being alive.

I discovered, almost by accident really, that allowing myself to feel sad, and to embrace that sadness, created a cathartic experience that stimulated me in a way that porn hadn't done for years. When I finally let myself feel the sadness, I had been neglecting myself for years, I felt an intense emotional rush, that seemed to set all of my neurons on fire. I sobbed alone in my room for about an hour. Just straight up ugly cried. Afterwards, I was left with an emotional high. It was not unlike the feeling post-orgasm, but much more powerful than I had ever experienced before.

By allowing myself to feel vulnerable, I realized that the feeling of release that came from orgasming, did not have to come from the act of masturbation alone. This was the moment I realized that porn didn't have to be the only thing that I had to feel. That I had the ability to feel something different, and that these feelings were more powerful and fulfilling than whatever cheap thrills masturbation provided. Even sadness felt so much more powerful and meaningful than the shallow excitement that came from my pornography addiction.

I may not ever be a perfect human being, but I know pretty damn well how to seek out what feels good, and for once I was ready to take a step in a different direction. This would end up being the very first step for me, and it may have only been a small one, but it was also essential for my recovery. Vulnerability had always been a tool used against me by my porn-addled addicted mind. The enemy knew exactly where to land the punch, but now I was the one that could wield it. Vulnerability had become a weapon for me to use to overcome the porn. Because now I was seeking a better feeling I possessed. Something pure that addiction couldn't corrupt.

I chased the feelings oozing out of my vulnerability like manna from the sky. The rewarding experience created by embracing my vulnerability made me want to seek it out again and again. Whenever I found myself getting emotional, I didn't automatically shut it out and distract myself with for porn and masturbation. Instead, I let the feelings I had suppressed for so long wash over me like rain. I allowed myself to feel sad and shitty. I stared long and hard into it, and found myself face to face with my shame, and once I had the courage to look it in the eye, I finally understood my enemy.

This was the first step of my addiction recovery and this will be one of the seven steps you will need to take to overcome yours. I put it as the first step because of how integral acceptance is to the effectiveness of your recovery. Without the ability to assess yourself and your feelings, you will not be able to understand what thoughts and actions are most beneficial to your fight against addiction. When you are able to be real with yourself, and willing to take a long hard look at yourself in the mirror, you can finally understand how your addiction works. When you understand why you became addicted and fell into these destructive habits in the first place, then you can also learn which thoughts and behaviors should be countered and avoided in the future.

For me, it took a long time to figure this out. Even after recognizing my addiction, I was not ready to understand it. I saw that it was there, that it was pulling me down further, but I was too scared and ashamed to figure out how to stop it. There was a period of several years where I would go through periods of trying to stop, trying to change my behaviors (see step 4) but because I wasn't willing to understand how I needed to change those behaviors, or what mentalities (see step 5) that I needed to revise to help my recovery along.

So, without that foundation of understanding my addiction to pornography, it would always be a case of two steps forward and two steps back. Getting real with my addiction, made me treat it with the respect it deserved. It had thoroughly and completely wrecked me, so I understood that it had to be treated as a legitimate enemy and threat. This would prove to be a pivotal step that led to later success down the road, as it gave me a resilient mentality. I understood how deep I was, but I could finally see the light emanating from the surface. I was ready to start climbing out of that hole.

If I could've handled my addiction recovery differently, it would have been to take this step much sooner. Ultimately, it was through gradual bouts of self-reflection and quasi-meditation practices which helped me come to terms with my addiction. Some people can figure this out on their own rather quickly, but for most (myself included) it can take a long time and a lot of additional struggle. For you, the smarter recovery, I would suggest you take this initial step much sooner. Seek out methods to help you uncover your vulnerabilities and discover the source of your addiction. Following guided meditations and self-reflections, even seeking out a therapist if that option is available to you. Your addiction spawns from a deep seeded issue in your life, and once you figure out what makes you tick, then you can start making serious headway with your addiction recovery.

6
STEP 2: EXPRESSING YOURSELF OUTWARDS

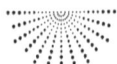

Seeking help from others is not only instrumental to you figuring out how your addiction works. Remember that your recovery is an uphill battle—a war even. Sometimes in war it is necessary to bring in reinforcements. You need allies to join you in your fight against addiction. This only becomes truer with a pornography addiction. The private nature of porn and masturbation makes it easy to keep your actions secret from your friends and family. If you grew up in a religious family, like I did, then you already know that admitting to this habit is akin to confessing your sins. I never felt comfortable expressing that I had a problem to my family because I knew that it would essentially be an admission of sin. Because of this, my addiction recovery became a cross that I had to bear alone, and I bore it for a long time.

Hiding my struggle didn't make my recovery any easier, and I wish that I had taken this step sooner in the process. It wasn't until I had found the No-Fap subreddit community on Reddit that I was finally able to start expressing my struggles outward. The anonymity of the online community made it easier for me to speak out about my struggles with pornography addiction, and even just typing out the different posts and comments in that community was therapeutic in a way. It was a small step, but a step in the right direction, and it was also occurring at the same time I was starting to open up to myself and pry into my own vulnerabilities. Taking small steps in both of these directions eventually gave me the first real foothold to help me claw my way out of the hole that was my pornography addiction.

Masturbation and my addiction to pornography were something that I always believed should be left unsaid, but interesting things start to happen once you push yourself to verbalize your thoughts and feelings about your addiction. Whenever I sat down to type out a post on the No-Fap community's subreddit, I had to engage in a kind of critical thinking that I was not used to. It felt bizarre, and extremely uncomfortable the first few times, but it was also another good exercise to get me to explore my vulnerabilities and really face my pornography addiction.

Even more beneficial was the kind of feedback I got from others whenever I put myself out there. The No-Fap community is one of those rare places on the internet where every interaction is positive, and all its anonymous members seem committed to genuinely helping each other out. I wasn't just getting one-or-two-word responses to my questions or comments. I was getting paragraphs of encouragement and valuable insight. Just knowing that I was being heard, and that there were people out there who understood what I was feeling was extremely helpful and affirming.

Through their support, and insight I felt empowered to change my habits and at least try to reprogram my mentality. I say the word "try" because alas I did try and failed. I was getting good advice from experienced members of the community, but I didn't fully understand the mechanics behind my addiction yet, so it was still a constant struggle. It wasn't until I was actively working on facing the truth behind my addiction (step 1) and engaging in the No-Fap community, that I started to see real progress with my addiction recovery.

The support and feedback I received from the anonymous online communities were an important early step to my recovery. Not only was I receiving good feedback and learning how to verbalize my addiction to others, but I was also introduced to the idea of accountability and making my recovery larger than myself. As silly as it may sound, I didn't want to disappoint these strangers who were being so kind in giving me their advice and encouragement. Accountability is huge in any type of addiction recovery and is the reason why so many people attend group sessions such as Alcoholics Anonymous.

Unfortunately, there are not many groups like this that meet strictly for pornography addiction, but as more and more fall into the trap of pornography in the future, I wouldn't be surprised in the slightest if public porn addiction support groups became more common. If you ever come across a group like this in your local community, I would strongly suggest taking this step as well. It is a good natural progression from completely anonymous online support groups and will be beneficial to help you externalize your pornography addiction and bring it further out into the light.

Externalization of your pornography addiction is perhaps the most essential component of step two. When you are able to verbalize and share your addiction with others, it can be a powerful tool in your fight against the addicted mind. Remember that your addicted mind wants you to feel alone and cutoff from the rest of the world. Opening up to others is just another way to open up yourself to the reality of your situation and allows others to chime in and give you even further perspective. The more you are able to open up about your addiction, the better foundation you are building for the many battles down the road. If there ever comes to be a moment of weakness or relapse, you will have a group of people you know you can fall back on. Having this support is essential for continuing to recover even after you face the inevitable relapse into the habit.

When choosing who to include in this so-called support group, you might be hesitant to include family and friends. This is what makes anonymous online and in-person groups more appealing to those who are still in the early phases of their pornography addiction recovery. You might have feelings of shame or embarrassment still in the forefront of your mind, holding you back from fully indulging your personal weakness and struggles with your friends and family. This is completely understandable, and there is by no means any rush to try and bring those closest to you in on your struggles with pornography and addiction

However, there will be a time when their inclusion will be necessary. Having anonymous support groups is great, and those groups can be very effective up to a certain point, but the only way to ensure that your addiction is thoroughly addressed, is by letting the people who really matter in your life in on your struggle and journey. For me, this came when I finally was able to share my struggle with addiction with my two of my close friends. My friends had known me since I first began college. They came into my life right when my addiction to pornography was advancing, but I still did not believe, or want to believe, that I had a problem. This was the era of my life when I was still sociable and dating, and porn just felt like a recreational habit (that I was doing once or twice every single day.)

So, my friends knew me, even if they weren't fully aware of my addiction. They also saw first-hand my gradual slip away from the land of the living, as I became further entrenched in my depression and addiction. To them, they had no idea what was causing me to spend less and less time with them, even after they tried to reach out to support and help me. I felt pretty poorly whenever I finally shared with them the reason, years later, and after a long time of not contacting them at all. It hurt to see how much my private porn addiction was affecting them and their feelings. I had made them feel hurt and confused by my unexplained drifting away from them years ago. Hearing this made my addiction even more real to me, and I remember apologizing again and again.

Telling them was a difficult thing to do at the time. Admittedly, it took me a few times to finally get it out, as I had chickened out several times. I was so nervous and scared to finally talk about it to them about it. I thought they might laugh at me or make jokes and not take my affliction seriously. Even in the moments just before letting the words roll out of my mouth, I felt butterflies in my stomach and my heart rate doubled. But my friends didn't laugh, they listened. They asked me good questions and once again I was learning how to verbalize my addiction, but this time it felt hugely significant. Each word out of my mouth felt like a weight falling off of my shoulder, and in that moment, I was exposed to them, but it felt good to be seen and heard.

Telling my friends was a big step in my recovery, and I am so glad that I finally took that step. The relief I felt was immense, and now I had a small group of people who I met and saw regularly who would ask me how I was doing with my recovery. It was just like sharing with the No-Fap community, but everything was so much bigger. Their words meant more; their advice meant more. I felt more compelled to stick to the positive habits, and the sense of accountability was much stronger whenever I felt the temptation to relapse.

Over time, I would open up to other friends and even a few family members. When opening up, you should be conscious about who you are including in your support group. Not everyone in your family or friend group is going to be receptive or understanding to your struggles. There are still family members who I haven't told partly because of how staunchly religious they are, and also because I know that they are less likely to offer me support. Whoever you open up to about your addiction is completely up to you but understand that not everyone needs to know about your struggle. The goal of step 2 is about building a support group and gaining reinforcements for your battles against addiction. You want to build a winning team that is going to have your best interests in mind.

7
STEP 3: DEDICATING YOURSELF TO DETOX

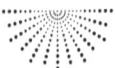

The third step to your recovery is probably the most straightforward. You need to stop masturbating to pornography. At this stage, you should be fully aware how serious your addiction has become. You are not at a stage where you can casually masturbate to pornography without feeding into this addictive behavior. The more you indulge in the habit, the longer it will persist, and the more difficult it will be to move your life into a more positive direction. So, quitting it not just a recommendation, it is essential.

How you go about quitting is something that is dependent on how deeply entrenched you are in your pornography addiction. Sometimes all it takes is the mentality to say "No." whenever the urge to masturbate presents itself, but if addiction has already warped your thoughts and behaviors, simply saying "No" might not be enough. So, there are several strategies you can use to help limit and reduce the temptation to masturbate. Not all will be effective for your particular situation, and if you haven't developed a strong foundation in steps 1 and 2, then you might be even harder pressed to successfully abstain and detox from your excessive masturbation habit.

For instance, one of the most direct ways you can keep yourself from indulging in pornography is by placing parental or website blockers on your personal computer. While this may seem like a patronizing was to handle your addiction, it can be extremely effective. For a long time, I tried to be strong and simply resist the urge to masturbate, but this would not always work, and eventually I would always end up on the same porn sites looking for a quick release. After I had finally opened up to some of my friends, I was able to use their help to keep myself accountable. I set a website blocker on my laptop and used their adult block feature to automatically filter out any sites or searches that could be considered pornographic. The only way I could turn off the website blocker was by entering a password, and the only person who knew that password was my friend.

This helped me out immensely, as it phased out my negative habit of masturbating to pornography, and I was able to limit the number of temptations I came across whenever I was using my personal laptop. It was the equivalent of me quitting cold turkey. I had drawn a line in the sand and decided I would not cross it. This is something we all must do in order to beat back addiction and reclaim our lives. Of course, quitting cold turkey is never easy. You will likely relapse a few times, like I did. But it is important to keep your mentality strong as you progress through your recovery. You need to keep pressing on even if you slip once or twice.

Withdrawals are difficult to deal with and can vary from person to person. While not as strong as the kind of withdrawals you may experience with alcohol or other substance driven addictions, withdrawal from porn and masturbation can still negatively impact the recovering addict. The reason why porn addicts can still experience the same withdrawals, is because you are creating an emotional muscle memory to the heightened feelings from masturbation. Every time you orgasm, your body releases a certain amount of dopamine to you mind.

Dopamine makes you feel good, and that heightened rush of emotion sends a fire throughout your brain, burning a hole in your memory. Do this to an excessive degree, and suddenly the fire is out of control, and it's the same pathways that are getting burned. Neurons in your head imploding over being over stimulated, and now your mind expects that burn. Withdrawal is the fire going out, and your body shakes because it thinks it needs that feeling again. Any of these feelings could happen to a porn addict who is trying to quit cold turkey. The main symptoms for me were more pronounced mood swings and a considerable lack of focus.

When I stopped dedicating so much time for porn, I realized that there was a lot of empty time in my schedule. Without knowing what to do with that time, I let my mind wander a bit and addressed some of the newfound questions I had for myself such as, *"Did I really free up this much of my schedule just so I could watch porn?"* and then I followed it up with, *"Are you really this much of a loser?"* These reoccurring negative thoughts made it difficult to successfully manage my newly found free time.

Besides the negative thoughts, I also found my body was affected by the sudden lack of porn. It was like my brain was on a daily dopamine diet, and as soon as I stopped masturbating, it cut off the supply. My brain grew furious at the body for not giving it its daily dose. My head demanded more of it. This left me feeling agitated and antsy all the time. I couldn't focus on tasks because there was always that nagging feeling of something, I should be providing for myself, but wasn't. Porn had literally hijacked my brain.

Of course, the withdrawals were hard on me whenever I tried to quit cold turkey. There were several times where the physical impulse alone caused me to relapse and feed that physical desire for release. At the time I would always feel terrible, but in retrospect I recognize how great my enemy was. Porn warped the physical mapping of my brain, rewiring it to expect a similar stimulation ever so often. Porn was changing me on a cellular level and that just goes to show how serious the addiction really is.

What your body and mind really need is a time to reset and heal, and quitting cold turkey is the best way to detox yourself from porn. The more space you give between orgasms, the less your mind will be guided by these impulses. When your brain is no longer demanding or expecting a hit of sexual stimulation, you can finally give yourself a chance to explore different kinds of stimulation. After an enough detox, your body will begin to recognize other kinds of stimulation, which means you finally give yourself a chance to change your habits and change your life.

8

STEP 4: RECONSTRUCT YOUR DAILY ROUTINE

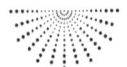

After detoxing from masturbation and being left with a considerable amount of energy and time at your disposal, you are now faced with several interesting choices. Before, you were resigned to the same old routine and habits, but now you have a chance to do something to make your life better. So, what is it going to be?

Every recovering addict will face this feeling eventually. Once you give yourself the chance to start thinking of a life without your crippling addiction weighing you down, you realize you actually have an opportunity to do something good and meaningful for yourself. The best way, and the most comprehensive way to approach these new sets of choices, is by consciously carving yourself a path. Before, your porn addiction was a set of repeating choices that kept you on the same path. But now, you finally have a chance to give your life a new direction. The secret is by replacing your negative habits and routines with positive ones.

Positive behaviors are the ones that are going to carry you a good portion of the way down the path of recovery. The more good you do for yourself and others, the more it will motivate your recovery to go onwards. Positive actions reap positive rewards, and the stimulation you receive from living your best life and being your best self will always come in a notch above any stimulation you have ever received from porn.

What these positive behaviors should resemble rests entirely on the innate needs of the addict. Porn was fulfilling a specific need for you, and that feeling was more than likely just a moment to feel good about yourself. To feel some relief, some sense of accomplishment. Porn is serving your needs in some way, however going about it in a negative, self-destructive way. The catch is, that just because masturbating to porn is a negative habit, it doesn't invalidate that base need of feeling good.

So, you need to discover what it is that you're missing. You need to know what need your porn is fulfilling. Once you recognize what purpose your masturbation is really trying to fulfill, you can replace that negative behavior with a positive one that fulfills the same purpose. You need to take stock in what actions and behaviors really matter to you. What is it that truly makes you happy, and what kind of good works can you do to make it happen?

A big behavior that I had to change during my addiction recovery was to finally take care of myself. When I was deepest into my pit of excess, I had let all the other areas of my life go to absolute shit. I didn't care what kind of foods that I ate, or how much I drank and smoke. I didn't care to shower, or bathe, or shave. I didn't go to bed at a reasonable time, I never exercised, and I only ever interacted with people if I absolutely had to. I wasn't taking care of myself. And it was having a serious impact on the quality of my life. When I was the most addicted to porn, I couldn't have cared less about the rest of my life because porn was all there was in my eyes. The highlight of my day had become my sad little buildup to orgasm.

After feeling fed up and disappointed with my past self, I decided to use these negative feelings and put them to good work. I used my frustration with myself to motivate me to do better, and to change my habits. So instead of giving in and jerking off, I would do a chore, or mark something off my to do list. I started viewing my life as a series of opportunities for decision-making. Your decisions can impact you in different ways. Some will make you feel good right away, but others take more time. The decisions that provide the most overall good for you and your future self, are the ones you should be making. Pornography is a short term means to an even shorter end. A single orgasm will never replace the utility of any task that will actually benefit your future.

Realizing this helped motivate me to take more conscientious actions. Instead of blowing a couple of hours away for a few seconds of orgasm, I could spend 20 minutes doing a task that could make my life a million times easier down the road. You should encourage any kind of thoughts you may have that aim to make better use of your time. In fact, I recommend you try keeping a daily planner just so you can see how much you can really do in the time it would normally take to maintain your porn habit. when you rewrite your daily behaviors, it's like you're reprogramming your porn-hacked brain. The secret is to fill your schedule with positive actions, and try to complete as many as possible,

I always would feel so fulfilled after seeing how much I was able to get done in the day. It felt so good, that I even pushed myself to be even more productive during in my days. My brain was craving it in a similar way that it would crave porn, and by fulfilling that need, I was giving myself the same kind of dopamine hit my body expected from porn. Only now, I was getting it from a positive habit that was actually helping to progress my life in a better direction. What makes this method of keeping a routine even more effective than porn, is how routines can help amplify the positive feelings over time, as opposed to making you eventually become numb to the sensation.

Whenever you complete a positive behavior, such as cleaning the house, or brushing your teeth, or going on a jog, or going to bed at a reasonable time—you are making things better for your future self. And in that future moment, when you realize how you are benefitting from something that your past-self had laid out for you, you begin to appreciate and love yourself even more. Something that pornography could never do in a million years.

9

STEP 5: REPROGRAM YOUR MENTALITY

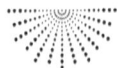

When you begin to change your physical behaviors, it will also begin to have an effect on your mind. For years I had to deal with the wall of insecurity that Porn had constructed around me and left me so detached from the world. Once I began to take positive actions that bettered my life, I began to feel things I had never felt before with porn. These feelings can sometimes be good, but they can also hurt. Even though you start to make the right choices in your life, you will always question whether or not you have the ability to maintain these positive changes.

When you are recovering from addiction, you begin to question yourself a lot. You recognize that you may be a flawed person, who is not living up to their potential, but you also have to put your mind in the right perspective. Making positive changes in your life is not about making yourself feel bad about who you are. You have to realize that changing is the sign of strength and growth, and you have to turn your recovery into your story.

I realized what my story was one random day. I was going through my daily planner, marking things off of my to do list, and feeling myself constantly thinking about how to set myself up for success, when I realized that what I was doing felt right. I felt okay about who I was and what I had done in the past. I embraced the fact that I may not have been the person I wanted to be, but that it was never too late for me to make the right kind of changes to turn that around.

As I became more in touch with my vulnerable feelings, I learned how to feel sympathy for my past self, instead of feeling the normal self-hatred and cynicism. It was so important for my recovery to have this thought process go through my head. I needed to find a way to mentally accept that I could change my ways and be a better person. I needed to believe that reality, and you will have to realize it as well. Without a positive mentality, you are likely to fall back into despair during your recovery. When despair creeps into your mind, it eventually will affect your habits, and bring your positive growth to a screeching halt. Despair opens the doors to relapsing into your pornography addiction. Whatever you do, do not give into despair.

Therefore, just like with your physical behaviors, you must learn how to replace your negative thoughts and feelings with ones that are more pleasant and optimistic. The more positive your mentality, the more positive your outlook will be for your recovery down the road. This means you need to take steps to help amplify positive feelings about yourself, your life, and your relationship with others. It's important to have time to affirm your own worth, and to see any signs of growth as a reason to keep pushing forward and fighting the good fight.

In addition to buying a daily planner, I also bought a daily journal. I used this journal to write down my personal thoughts and feelings. Doing this helped me get a good grasp on how my mentality was changing over time. I was able to take note whenever I was feeling motivated and excited, and also the times when I was feeling down and hopeless. Keeping daily entries helped me track how my mood changed between the two, and I soon discovered that my mood was following a pattern going up and down gradually over time like a sine graph.

Keeping a daily journal also helped me see the overall projection of my addiction recovery. looking back over the many pages of my journal reassured me that I was actually making progress in my overall recovery, and that while my feelings may rise and fall, my general mood was still moving in a positive direction. Having this method of charting my progress was hugely beneficial for my positive mentality. When you have the right mindset, you can truly overcome anything.

Positivity can come from many different directions. Once you begin to create positive routines for yourself, don't neglect saving time to do some things that will serve your mental health. Make sure to engage your mind during your recovery. Seek out ways to engage yourself emotionally, as well as creatively, and make sure to take note of the most positively rejuvenating moments so you can learn where and when to seek them out again.

The more negative thoughts and behaviors you replace with positive ones, the further along you will progress down the path of recovery. Remember that recovery is not an in and out process. It's not a two-week detox, or a whole month of rehabilitation. Recovery is a lifestyle, and something that you will have to engage in for the rest of your life. Steps 1 through 3 are designed to create a platform for you to build from, and steps 4 and 5 are designed to give you momentum as you carry on down the road to recovery. The next two steps are designed to make sure that you are able to sustain the long haul of your journey and are the final steps you must take to fully realize your addiction recovery.

10

STEP 6: ACCEPTING YOUR VICTORIES AND YOUR DEFEATS

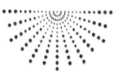

One of the hardest parts of any addiction recovery is admitting that you still have a long way to go. It can be hard to maintain a certain set of positive thoughts and behaviors if you are starting to feel like it is impossible to sustain your new habits. This cynical line of thinking is exactly the way Pornography can regain a hold on your life and work its way back into your mind. You begin to feel the temptation to rest on your laurels and give in to the feeling once more. After all, it's only taking a few steps back. Nothing wrong with that—eh. The answer is always no. It is never good to give in to the cynical feelings of "So what?"

Being cynical and hopeless will only drag you further down the path of an addict and only work to destroy the positive systems you have started to reintroduce into your life. There is nothing beneficial to viewing this recovery as a matter of success and failures. This is why I lean so heavily on the battle imagery when it comes to your addiction. It really is a fight. One of the biggest fights you might ever need to face in your life. This is you verses the addicted mind. One of the most cunning and conniving enemies you will ever face. When you remember that you are in the middle of self v self-warfare, you start to appreciate how difficult your situation truly is.

The fact that you are even wanting to face your addiction like this is a sign of your bravery. You may be up against tough odds, but as long as you keep pushing forward, you will always give yourself more opportunities to improve your life for the better. Your addiction earns a lot of respect. I mean, look what it has done to your life. You are right to want to turn the tide of battle and start taking the fight to your addiction. You may have a tough battle ahead, and you may very well be the underdog in this fight, but just like in the movies, everybody cheers for the underdog to win. You will definitely be cheering once you achieve your first victory.

Victories come in all shapes and sizes. Maybe you spent your first full 24-hours of not looking at porn. Maybe you haven't masturbated at all in a week. Maybe you just put on pants and went out with friends like this. There are so many different kinds of victories you can have on any given day. When you achieve even the smallest victory, it is important for you to take note. Be proud of your accomplishment and try to savor its memory.

For combatting my own shame, I needed these small moments of pride in myself to help push me on down the road of recovery. It became a kind of game that I wanted to win. I wanted to be very good at winning, so I pushed myself to win every single time, and as pride replaced shame, I was motivated to continue being the best version of myself that I could possibly be. Winning all of those little battles against my addiction gradually taught me that I was more than the sum parts of my addiction. I was a living breathing human being just like everyone else. And on some level, I deserved to be happy.

Part of getting real with yourself and learning reprogram your mentality leans heavily on the simple premise that you are someone that deserves to be happy. If you are anything like me, you will have a hard time accepting the new feelings of happiness and pride. You might reflect over the darkness of your past, or you feel unworthy of any kind of love and affection for how easily you were consumed by your addiction, but you need to fight these negative thoughts and feelings. You need to accept that you are capable and deserving of love, and that there is nothing that can take that away from you. Once you accept that you deserve to be happy, then you can really start treating your small victories as significant victories and feel motivated to keep pushing through the fight against your addicted mind.

Treating your addiction recovery like an ongoing battle will also lessen the sting of defeat whenever you inevitably relapse again. In my journey towards recovery, there were many setbacks. Most occurred in the early stages of recovery, but that doesn't mean that I was free from slipping up once I was a veteran of recovery. The truth is, that there might be a time after years of maintaining positive thoughts and behaviors that you still make a mistake.

Relapse can happen at any time. Sometimes it comes after lots of self-rationalizing and other times it can just be a whim. Relapse into pornography is especially easy because it doesn't take much for someone to suddenly react on the impulse to masturbate. With internet and social media, there are plenty of ways to entice the mind to take a detour and indulge in your old negative habit.

Whenever you fall short and give in to relapse, you should not consider it a personal failure, but an actual defeat at the hands of an enemy. When you frame your recovery in within this concept of having an oppositional force, you can be more forgiving towards yourself. You can work through the process in your mind, and explain to yourself that, "You are not a weak person, your addiction just got the better of you." Being more optimistic towards your progress in your fight against addiction will encourage you to keep engaging in positive thoughts and behavior instead of slipping back into masturbation.

As you weigh your victories against your defeats, you will start to understand how well your recovery has suited you. You will appreciate the tools that you gained from your various struggles and tough lessons learned. You will learn how to lean back on your progress down the road, and if you ever fall short from time to time, you can put that small defeat in the context of your entire battle with porn addiction. When you consider all of the victories you won in your fight against the addicted mind, you will feel good about how much improved your life is becoming, and the occasional relapse will not seem as bad.

11
STEP 7: ASSESS, ADDRESS, AND PRESS ON

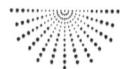

Remember where you were when you were at your absolute lowest. When you were caught up in the cycle of pornography and masturbation addiction. You were in shambles and your life had no meaning or direction. You were stuck, and because of that stillness you were letting the rest of the world pass you by as you folded in on yourself. You were a tangle of negative thoughts and feelings that swirled out of your pornography addiction, and you just sat idly by as it wreaked havoc on your life.

While you may despise the cycle that brought you so low, you should never pass up a learning moment. Even though it was a cycle that held you down, it doesn't mean that all cycles are bad. Your pornography addiction was a cycle that brought you down, but there is another cycle you must understand in order for you to successfully sustain your recovery.

I call this final step "Assess, Address, and Press On" because I believe these words best describe the positive cycle you must complete in order to keep your recovery going strong. Consider the what the antonyms of each three would be: "Ignore, Deny, and Retreat." These inverted words perfectly encapsulate the cycle behind your addiction. You start by ignoring your problem, denying the feelings behind your addiction, and finally by retreating back to the habits you have an unhealthy relationship with. If you can replace the negative cycle with the positive one, then you will always have a chance to progress your recovery.

You can consider steps 1 through 7 as the cycle of addiction recovery. Although you may not take each step linearly, they are all moving you down the path of recovery. Once you have made some progress on your recovery then you are ready to assess the progress you've made thus far, address any issues that you are currently facing, and then press on with the positive thoughts and behaviors that bring you closer to the person you want to be.

If you actively engage in Step 7 throughout your addiction recovery, then you allow yourself to go back into the cycle with direction and a purpose. Once you've assessed your progress, then you can see all the areas where you've grown as a person. Taking the time to read through past journals or planners and see the positive differences in your behaviors overtime can really boost your confidence and motivation to continue. You will gain this healthy image of yourself and develop a deeper belief that you have the capability to keep growing into the person you want to be.

When you assess your progress, you can also analyze areas where you could improve. No recovery happens flawlessly, and you will always find yourself caught in moments of weakness. Once you understand the mentality of war and accept that your mistakes are just lessons for the next battle, then you can learn from the defeats you suffered at the hands of your addiction. Now you can recognize which behaviors and thoughts are becoming the most productive in terms of your recovery and which thoughts and behaviors should be avoided in the future.

When you address your shortcomings, you have the opportunity to make good the thoughts and behaviors the next time they come around again. Because recovery is a cycle, it means you will always have the chance to try again. If you relapse for the first time in over a month, you still have the chance to come back and abstain for two months more. Addressing where you made a mistake, or felt a relapse was imminent, then you can double your efforts to avoid the thoughts and behaviors that lead you towards defeat.

After you have assessed and addressed your recovery, then you are ready to continue the cycle. You are ready to press on. And you should keep pressing ahead even when you don't feel as motivated to carry on. There will be times when you feel discouraged or even straight up apathetic— and if you do, you're still okay. It's okay to struggle with your addiction recovery. It is a war after all, and it hasn't been easy.

Continuing the cycle of recovery will provide you with sustainable growth. This is the only way to ensure that your lifestyle always remains on the path of recovery, and keep the negative structures brought on by addiction at bay. It may be difficult to know when a good time is to reflect over your addiction recovery, since steps 1 through 6 happen so irregularly. The key for gaining the most insight is by reflecting over periods where you have noted a change. Analyze what that change is and what it means to you. Are you feeling better about who you are and what you bring to the world? Are you feeling more at home with your friends and at your job? Do you feel yourself brimming with purpose and fulfillment?

Assessing, addressing, and pressing on will always be essential steps towards your recovery. The better you understand yourself and how you move down the paths of addiction and recovery, the more control you will have on where you lie on those different paths. When you feel yourself achieving growth in cycle after cycle, then you know you are truly winning the war against your addiction and that you are finally approaching the best version of yourself to date.

AFTERWORD

Much like the first time you realized you were addicted to pornography, the realization that you are recovered will happen after a while, and totally catch you by surprise. One day you will wake up and the seven steps will all seem so natural to you. You will be set in a routine of positive behaviors that bring your life happiness and fulfillment. You will find yourself with a better outlook on your future, and the thrill of new challenges and bigger decisions. You will feel confident in yourself and in your ability to maintain this best version of yourself.

Eventually after years of feeling this way, after becoming comfortable in your skin, and accepting of who you are and who you were, you will begin to allow yourself to admit that you are better now. That you have recovered a big chunk of your life back from your addiction and now you are truly living. You won't always think back to those dark days, but whenever you do you will find comfort knowing that you are a different person on a different course now. You will see that person as a mere snapshot of you stretched out over the spectrum of your life.

AFTERWORD

Once you start taking all seven steps, you will make some serious headway down your road to recovery. Just remember that even the smallest step forward is something worth celebrating, and that you are only setting yourself up for a better future tomorrow. There will be plenty of challenges and learning moments ahead for you. But you are more than capable of overcoming them and rising above. You are stronger than you think, and you should be proud of yourself for taking the bold first steps in a new direction.

What's waiting for you on the other side of addiction is a life full of promise and potential. A world that is not overrun by cheap momentary thrills, but a world that governed by great slow burning feelings. You will finally find love in the world, and not just from someone else, bur love that you find for yourself. Love that makes you feel like you have a place and purpose in the world. Love that wakes you up in the morning and tucks you back in at night. You have a life full of love to look forward to, and love coming from all directions.

I can't wait to meet you there on the other side, in your new life of slow-burning love. When you face the inevitable hardships, just remember what's there waiting for you and find the resilience to carry on. Resilience will keep you during the toughest moments of recovery. Don't forget to lean on your community for support when things get too heavy, and never stop filling your life with positive thoughts, feelings and actions. Understand that everyone will carve their own path out of their addiction, and you will eventually find your own. Carry on and keep fighting the good fight. I hope that you overcome that pit of excess in your life and I wish you all the best of luck as you go about your addiction recovery.

Thank you for making it through to the end of *Pornog-*

AFTERWORD

raphy and Masturbation Addiction Mastery, let's hope it was informative and able to provide you with all of the tools you need to achieve your goals, whatever they may be.

www.ingramcontent.com/pod-product-compliance
Lightning Source LLC
Chambersburg PA
CBHW021451070526
44577CB00002B/354